Intern

Fasting Cookbook

for Everyone

Discover The Lastest Cookbook for Beginners To Lose Weight and Stay Fit With Amazing Recipes.

Sam Donno

Additionally, the information in the following pages is intended only for informational purposes and should thus be thought of as universal. As befitting its nature, it is presented without assurance regarding its prolonged validity or interim quality. Trademarks that are mentioned are done without written consent and can in no way be considered an endorsement from the trademark holder.

Table of Contents

BREAKFAST

1. Bacon Hash

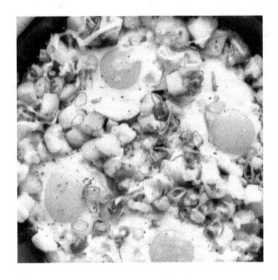

Preparation Time: 5 minutes

Cooking Time: 10 minutes

Servings: 2

Ingredients:

- Small green pepper (1)
- Jalapenos (2)
- Small onion (1)

- Eggs (4)
- Bacon slices (6)

Directions:

1. Chop the bacon into chunks using a food processor. Set aside for now. Slice the onions and peppers into thin strips. Dice the jalapenos as small as possible.
2. Heat a skillet and fry the veggies. Once browned, combine the fixings and cook until crispy. Place on a serving dish with the eggs.

Nutrition: Carbohydrates: 9 grams Protein: 23 grams Fats: 24 grams Calories: 366

2. Bagels with Cheese

Preparation Time: 10 minutes

Cooking Time: 15 minutes

Servings: 6

Ingredients:

- Mozzarella cheese (2.5 cups)
- Baking powder (1 tsp.)
- Cream cheese (3 oz.)
- Almond flour (1.5 cups)
- Eggs (2)

Directions:

1. Shred the mozzarella and combine with the flour, baking powder, and cream cheese in a mixing container. Pop into the microwave for about one minute. Mix well.
2. Let the mixture cool and add the eggs. Break apart into six sections and shape into round bagels. Note: You can also sprinkle with a

seasoning of your choice or pinch of salt if desired.

3. Bake them for approximately 12 to 15 minutes. Serve or cool and store.

Nutrition: Carbohydrates: 8 grams Protein: 19 grams Fats: 31 grams Calories: 374

3. Cauli Flitters

Preparation Time: 10 minutes

Cooking Time: 15 minutes

Servings: 2

Ingredients:

- 2 eggs
- 1 head of cauliflower
- 1 tbsp. yeast
- sea salt, black pepper
- 1-2 tbsp. ghee
- 1 tbsp. turmeric
- 2/3 cup almond flour

Directions:

1. Place the cauliflower into a large pot and start to boil it for 8 mins. Add the florets into a food processor and pulse them.
2. Add the eggs, almond flour, yeast, turmeric, salt and pepper to a mixing bowl. Stir well. Form into patties.

3. Heat your ghee to medium in a skillet. Form your fritters and cook until golden on each side (3-4 mins).
4. Serve it while hot.

Nutrition: Calories: 238 kcal Fat: 23 g Carbs: 5 g Protein: 6 g

4. Scrambled Eggs

Preparation Time: 2 minutes

Cooking Time: 8 minutes

Servings: 4

Ingredients:

- 4 oz. butter
- 8 eggs
- salt and pepper for taste

Directions:

1. Crack the eggs in a bowl, and whisk them together, while seasoning it.
2. Melt the butter in a skillet over medium heat, but don't turn it into brown.
3. Pour the eggs into the skillet and cook it for 1-2 mins, until they look and feel fluffy and creamy.
4. Tip: If you want to shake things up, you can pair this one up with bacon, salmon, or maybe avocado as well.

Nutrition: Carbs: 1 g Fat: 31 g Protein: 11 g Calories: 327 kcal

5. Frittata with Spinach

Preparation Time: 5 minutes

Cooking Time: 30 minutes

Servings: 4

Ingredients:

- 8 eggs
- 8 ozs. fresh spinach
- 5 ozs. diced bacon
- 5 ozs. shredded cheese
- 1 cup heavy whipping cream
- 2 tbsps. butter
- salt and pepper

Directions:

1. Preheat the oven to 350 °F
2. Fry the bacon until crispy, add the spinach and cook until wilted. Set them aside.
3. Whisk the cream and eggs together, and pour it into the baking dish.

4. Add the cheese, spinach, and bacon on the top, and place in the oven. Bake for 25-30 minutes, until golden brown on top.

Nutrition: Carbs: 4 g Fat: 59 g Protein: 27 g Calories: 661 kcal

6. Cheese Omelet

Preparation Time: 5 minutes

Cooking Time: 10 minutes

Servings: 2

Ingredients:

- 6 eggs
- 3 ozs. ghee
- 7 ozs. shredded cheddar cheese
- salt and pepper

Directions:

1. Whisk the eggs until smooth. Compound half of the cheese and season it with salt and pepper.
2. Melt the butter in a pan. Pour in the mixture and let it sit for a few minutes (3-4)
3. When the mixture is looking good, add the other half of the cheese. Serve immediately.

Nutrition: Carbs: 4 g Fat: 80 g Protein: 40 g Calories: 897 kcal

7. Capicola Egg Cups

Preparation Time: 5 minutes

Cooking Time: 15 minutes

Servings: 4

Ingredients:

- 8 eggs
- 1 cup cheddar cheese
- 4 oz. capicola or bacon (slices)
- salt, pepper, basil

Directions:

1. Preheat the oven to 400°F. You will need 8 wells of a standard-size muffin pan.
2. Place the slices in the 8 wells, forming a cup shape. Sprinkle into each cup some of the cheese, according to your liking.
3. Crack an egg into each cup, season them with salt and pepper.
4. Bake for 10-15 mins. Serve hot, top it with basil.

Nutrition: Carbs: 1 g Fat: 11 g Protein: 16 g Calories: 171 kcal

8.   Overnight "noats"

Preparation Time: 5 minutes plus overnight to chill

Cooking Time: 10 minutes

Servings: 1

Ingredients:

- 2 tablespoons hulled hemp seeds
- 1 tablespoon chia seeds
- ½ scoop (about 8 grams) collagen powder
- ½ cup unsweetened nut or seed milk (hemp, almond, coconut, and cashew)

Direction:

1. In a small mason jar or glass container, combine the hemp seeds, chia seeds, collagen, and milk.
2. Secure tightly with a lid, shake well, and refrigerate overnight.

Nutrition: Calories: 263 Total Fat: 19g Protein: 16g Total Carbs: 7g Fiber: 5g Net Carbs: 2g

LUNCH

9. Colorful Chicken Casserole

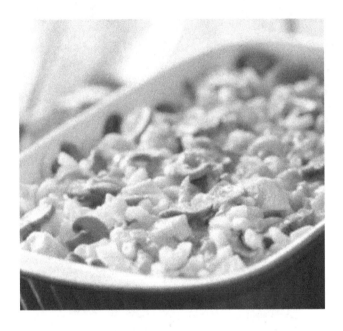

Preparation Time: 14 minutes

Cooking Time: 14 minutes

Servings: 6

Ingredients:

- 1 cup broth, chicken
- 3 cups cooked chicken, diced

- 4 cups chopped broccoli
- 1 cup assorted colored bell peppers, chopped
- 1 cup cream
- 4 T sherry
- ¼ c hand-shredded Parmesan cheese
- 1 small size can black olives, sliced, drained
- 2 Tortilla Factory low-carb whole wheat tortillas
- ½ c hand-shredded mozzarella

Directions:

1. Place broccoli and chicken broth into a skillet.
2. Top with lid, bring to a boil, and steam until desired crispness. (4 min)
3. Add the peppers, steam for one minute if you don't want them crisp.
4. Add the chicken and stir to heat.
5. Combine the sherry, cream, parmesan, and olives.
6. Tear the tortillas into bite-sized pieces.
7. Stir into the chicken and broccoli.
8. Pour cream sauce over the chicken, stir.
9. Top with hand-shredded mozzarella.

10.   Broil in oven until cheese is melted and golden brown.

Nutrition: Calories: 412 Total Fat: 30g Protein: 29 Total Carbs: 10g Dietary Fiber: 9g Sugar: 1g Sodium: 712mg

10. Chicken Relleno Casserole

Preparation Time: 19 minutes

Cooking Time: 29 minutes

Servings: 6

Ingredients:

- 6 Tortilla Factory low-carb whole wheat tortillas, torn into small pieces
- 1 ½ cups hand-shredded cheese, Mexican
- 1 beaten egg
- 1 cup milk
- 2 cups cooked chicken, shredded
- 1 can Ro-tel
- ½ cup salsa Verde

Directions:

1. Grease an 8 x 8 glass baking dish
2. Heat oven to 375 degrees
3. Combine everything together, but reserve ½ cup of the cheese
4. Bake it for 29 minutes

5. Take it out of oven and add ½ cup cheese

6. Broil for about 2 minutes to melt the cheese

Nutrition: Calories: 265 Total Fat: 16gProtein: 20g Total Carbs: 18g Dietary Fiber: 10g Sugar: 0g Sodium: 708mg

11. Italian Chicken with Asparagus and Artichoke Hearts

Preparation Time: 9 minutes

Cooking Time: 40 minutes

Servings: 1

Ingredients:

- 1 can long asparagus spears, drained
- 1 c red peppers, roasted, drained
- 1 c artichoke hearts, drained
- 6 oz. of boneless chicken breast, pounded thin or sliced thinly
- 2 T parmesan cheese
- 1 T Bisquick
- ½ tsp oregano
- ½ tsp garlic powder
- ½ cup fresh sliced mushrooms
- 2 T red wine vinegar
- 2 T butter
- 3 T olive oil

Directions:

1. Place in a small blender container (or bowl) the oregano, garlic powder, vinegar, and 1 T oil. Place to the side.
2. Combine the Bisquick and Parmesan cheese.
3. Roll the chicken in the Bisquick and Parmesan mix.
4. Heat the butter in a skillet.
5. Brown the chicken on both sides and cook until done, approximately 4 minutes.
6. Emulsify or quickly whip the wet ingredients you have placed to the side. This is your dressing.
7. Place the chicken on the plate.
8. Surround with the vegetables and drizzle them with the dressing.

Nutrition: Calories: 435 Total Fat: 18g Protein: 38g Total Carbs: 16g Dietary Fiber: 7g Sugar: 1g Sodium: 860mg

12. Kabobs with Peanut Curry Sauce

Preparation Time: 9 minutes

Cooking Time: 9 minutes

Servings: 4

Ingredients:

- 1 cup Cream
- 4 tsp Curry Powder
- 1 1/2 tsp Cumin
- 1 1/2 tsp Salt
- 1 T minced garlic
- 1/3 cup Peanut Butter, sugar-free
- 2 T Lime Juice
- 3 T Water
- 1/2 small Onion, diced
- 2 T Soy Sauce
- 1 packet Splenda
- 8 oz. boneless, cooked Chicken Breast
- 8 oz. pork tenderloin

Directions:

1. Blend together cream, onion, 2 tsp. garlic, curry and cumin powder, and salt.
2. Slice the meats into 1-inch pieces.
3. Place the cream sauce into a bowl and put in the chicken and tenderloin to marinate. Let rest in sauce for 14 minutes.
4. Blend peanut butter, water, 1 tsp. garlic, lime juice, soy sauce, and Splenda. This is your peanut dipping sauce.
5. Remove the meats and thread on skewers. Broil or grill 4 minutes per side until meat is done.
6. Serve with dipping sauce.

Nutrition: Calories: 530 Total Fat: 29g Protein: 37g Total Carbs: 6g Dietary Fiber: 4g Sugar: 2g Sodium: 1538mg

13. Pizza

Preparation Time: 4 minutes

Cooking Time: 4 minutes

Servings: 1

Ingredients:

- 1 Tortilla Factory low carb whole wheat tortilla
- ¼ cup mozzarella cheese, hand-shredded
- ¼ cup tomato paste
- sprinkle of Italian seasoning
- sprinkle of garlic salt
- Cut the broccoli, spinach, mushrooms, peppers, and onions you like for toppings

Directions:

1. Turn broiler on in oven, or toaster oven
2. Spread tortilla with tomato paste
3. Sprinkle seasoning on the paste
4. Add the cheese
5. Add the veggies

6. Broil or toast 1-4 minutes until crust is crunchy and cheese melted

Nutrition: Calories: 155 Total Fat: 7g Protein: 13g Total Carbs: 18g Dietary Fiber: 10g Sugar: 2g Sodium: 741mg

14. Salmon with Bok-Choy

Preparation Time: 9 minutes

Cooking Time: 9 minutes

Servings: 4

Ingredients:

- 1 c red peppers, roasted, drained
- 2 cups chopped bok-choy
- 1 T salted butter
- 5 oz. salmon steak
- 1 lemon, sliced very thinly
- 1/8 tsp black pepper
- 1 T olive oil
- 2 T sriracha sauce

Directions:

1. Place oil in skillet
2. Place all but 4 slices of lemon in the skillet.
3. Sprinkle the bok choy with the black pepper.
4. Stir fry the bok-choy with the lemons.
5. Remove and place on four plates.

6. Place the butter in the skillet and stir fry the salmon, turning once.

7. Place the salmon on the bed of bok-choy.

8. Divide the red peppers and encircle the salmon.

9. Place a slice of lemon atop the salmon.

10. Drizzle with sriracha sauce.

Nutrition: Calories: 410 Total Fat: 30g Protein: 30g Total Carbs: 7g Dietary Fiber: 2g Sugar: 0g Sodium: 200mg

15. Sriracha Tuna Kabobs

Preparation Time: 4 minutes

Cooking Time: 9 minutes

Servings: 4

Ingredients:

- 4 T Huy Fong chili garlic sauce
- 1 T sesame oil infused with garlic
- 1 T ginger, fresh, grated
- 1 T garlic, minced
- 1 red onion, cut into quarters and separated by petals
- 2 cups bell peppers, red, green, yellow
- 1 can whole water chestnuts, cut in half
- ½ pound fresh mushrooms, halved
- 32 oz. boneless tuna, chunks or steaks
- 1 Splenda packet
- 2 zucchini, sliced 1 inch thick, keep skins on

Directions:

1. Layer the tuna and the vegetable pieces evenly onto 8 skewers.

2. Combine the spices and the oil and chili sauce, add the Splenda

3. Quickly blend, either in blender or by quickly whipping.

4. Brush onto the kabob pieces, make sure every piece is coated

5. Grill 4 minutes on each side, check to ensure the tuna is cooked to taste.

6. Serving size is two skewers.

Nutrition: Calories: 467 Total Fat: 18g Protein: 56g Total Carbs: 21g   Dietary Fiber: 3.5g Sugar: 6g Sodium: 433mg

DINNER

16. Colombian Steak with Onions and Tomatoes

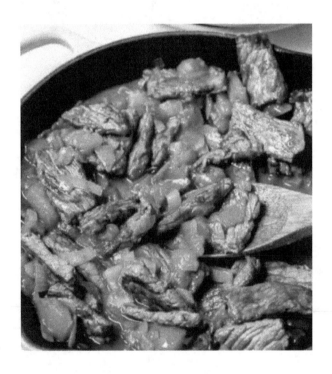

Preparation Time: 10 minutes

Cooking Time: 50 minutes

Servings: 6

Ingredients

- 1½ lbs. grass-fed sirloin tip steak, sliced thinly
- 1 medium onion, sliced or chopped thinly
- 1 large tomato (or 2 medium tomatoes), sliced or chopped thinly
- 4 tsps. olive oil, divided
- Garlic powder
- Cumin
- Salt

Directions

1. Season the steak with garlic powder and salt.
2. Place a large skillet over high heat. Add 2 tbsps. of oil and heat. Working in batches, cook the first half of the steak about 1 minute. Stir halfway to cook evenly. Once cooked, transfer to a plate. Do this step to the remaining batch then set aside?
3. Reduce the heat to medium. Using the same pan, heat oil and sauté the onions for 2 minutes. Add the tomatoes and season with cumin, salt, and pepper. Reduce heat to medium-low.

4. Add about a quarter cup of water and let simmer for a few minutes to reduce the liquid volume. Add more water if needed and adjust the taste accordingly.
5. Return the steak to the skillet with its drippings. Mix well before removing the pan from the heat.
6. Serve with rice or a fried egg on top.

Nutrition: calories378, fat 8g, fiber 2g, carbs 8g, protein 6g

17. Maple Walnut-Glazed Black-Eyed Peas with Collard Greens

Preparation Time: 10 minutes

Cooking Time: 30 minutes

Servings: 3

Ingredients

For the maple-walnut glaze:

- ¾ cup water
- ½ cup walnuts, chopped
- ½ tbsp. Tamari sauce
- 2 tbsps. sugar-free maple syrup
- 1 tsp. arrowroot starch flour
- Dash of nutmeg
- ½ tsp. ground mustard
- ⅛ tsp. ground ginger
- ⅛ tsp. ground cinnamon
- ⅛ tsp. ground cloves
- For the black-eyed peas and collard greens
- 4 cups cooked black-eyed peas

- 1 large bunch fresh collard greens, cleaned, stems removed, and chopped
- ¼ cup water (plus more)

Directions

1. For the maple-walnut glaze, put all ingredients in a blender in this order: water, walnuts, tamari, maple syrup, starch, and the spices. Blend starting at the lowest setting and gradually adjust to the highest. Blend on high about 40 seconds. Set aside.

2. For the peas and collards, place a 5-quart sauté pan over medium-high heat and add water. Put the collards and steam-sauté until tender, about 10 minutes. You can also adjust the doneness according to your preference.

3. Add the glaze to the greens and continue to cook on medium-high about 2 minutes. Stir frequently.

4. Add the peas. Continue to cook and stir another minute. Serve immediately.

Nutrition: calories 233, fat 8g, fiber 2g, carbs 8g, protein 13g

18. Garlic Shrimp with Zucchini Noodles

Preparation Time: 10 minutes

Cooking Time: 4 minutes

Servings: 3

Ingredients

- 1 lb. shrimp, shelled and deveined
- 2 medium zucchini, spiraled
- 2 tbsps. fresh chives, minced
- 2 tbsps. fresh lemon juice
- 4 garlic cloves, minced
- 2 tbsps. coconut oil
- Sea salt
- Freshly ground black pepper

Directions

1. Place a skillet over medium heat and heat the oil.
2. Sauté the garlic about 2-3 minutes.
3. Add the shrimp and cook2-4 minutes or until pink. Remove the shrimp from the pan.

4. Add the lemon juice and stir. Bring the mixture to a boil and simmer until most of the liquid has evaporated.

5. Mix in the zucchini noodles and continue to cook another 3-4 minutes.

6. Bring the shrimp back to the skillet and season to taste. Stir well and sprinkle with chives before serving.

Nutrition: calories 280, fat 8g, fiber 3g, carbs 8g, protein 6g

19. Vietnamese Turkey Meatball Bowls

Preparation Time: 10 minutes

Cooking Time: 30 minutes

Servings: 3

Ingredients

- For the meatballs
- 1 lb. ground turkey
- ¼ cup coconut oil
- 0.4 oz. (or 1-inch) piece fresh ginger, minced
- 2 garlic cloves, minced
- 1 tsp. fish sauce
- 1 tsp. tamari
- ¼tsp. sea salt
- ¼ tsp. white pepper

For the quick pickles

- 1 cup cucumber, sliced into thin rounds
- 4 radishes, thinly sliced
- ½ cup carrots, cut into matchsticks

- 2 tbsps. rice wine vinegar
- 2 tbsps. water
- Pinch of red pepper flakes
- For the toppings
- 3.5 oz. shirataki noodles
- 2 Lime wedges
- Mixed herbs (like Thai basil, mint, cilantro)

Directions

1. For the meatballs, mixed all ingredients in a medium-size mixing bowl and make 2-inch balls.
2. Place a large skillet over medium-high heat and heat oil. Cook the meatballs about 3-4 minutes per side until cooked through.
3. For the pickles, combine all ingredients in a small bowl.
4. Prepare the shirataki noodles according to package instructions.
5. To serve, divide the noodles, turkey meatballs, and pickles between 2 bowls. Garnish with herbs and a lime wedge.

Nutrition: calories 170, Fat 5g, Protein 8g, Carbs 7g

20. Filipino Chicken Adobo

Preparation Time: 10 minutes

Cooking Time: 20 minutes

Servings: 4

Ingredients

- 1 lb. boneless chicken, cut into pieces
- 2 tbsps. Soy sauce
- 3 tbsps. Apple cider vinegar
- 1½ tsps. Garlic, minced
- 2 tbsps. Olive oil

Directions

1. Mix the soy sauce, vinegar, garlic, and oil in a pan.
2. Add the chicken and coat it with the soy sauce mixture.
3. Place the pan over medium heat, add the chicken, cover with a lid, and let it simmer 10-15 minutes.

4. Uncover the pan and adjust the heat to medium-high. Cook until the chicken is browned. Stir occasionally to avoid burning.

5. Serve and enjoy!

Nutrition: calories 207, fat 8g, fiber 2g, carbs 8g, protein 6g

21. Kale & Artichoke Soup

Preparation Time: 10 minutes

Cooking Time: 30 minutes

Servings: 3

Ingredients

- 2 cups artichoke hearts*
- 2 cups kale leaves, tightly packed and stem discarded
- 32 oz. low sodium chicken broth
- ½ white sweet potato, chopped into ½-inch slices
- 1 cup unsweetened almond milk
- 1 large yellow onion, chopped
- 1 pinch cayenne pepper
- 1 pinch ground nutmeg
- 2 tbsps. olive oil
- Sea salt

Directions

1. Place a pot over medium heat and heat the oil. Sauté the onions about 8-10 minutes or until translucent.
2. Put in the sweet potatoes and continue to cook, stirring frequently, until soft.
3. Add the artichoke hearts, broth, nutmeg, and cayenne. Season with salt and bring to a boil.
4. Lower the heat and simmer 10 minutes.
5. Add the kale and cover the pot with a lid. Leave it for a minute until the kale leaves have wilted.
6. Add the almond milk. Next, using an immersion blender, process the mixture until smooth. Alternatively, transfer the soup to the blender and process in batches.
7. Strain the soup to separate the strands of artichoke hearts. Serve the soup hot or cold.
8. Drizzle with oil before serving.

Nutrition: calories 108, fat 8g, fiber 2g, carbs 8g, protein 7g

22. Poached Eggs and Bacon on Toast

Preparation Time: 10 minutes

Cooking Time: 30 minutes

Servings: 1

Ingredients

- Bacon 2 slices
- Eggs 2 medium
- Salmon (If you want)
- Spinach baby leaf 200 grams
- Black pepper
- Sea salt
- Toast 1 slice

Direction

1. Make a large pan of water to a gentle boil.
2. Stir the water gently and then break the eggs; poach for 4 minutes or until the whites are set.

3. During that time, heat a deep-frying pan, add a splash of water, and sprinkle with the spinach. Cook for 2 minutes until the mixture is withered.

4. Take spinach and place it aside on a plate. Fry the bacon till golden brown.

5. Put the spinach (and salmon) on a toast, sprinkle with salt and pepper.

6. Cover all of it with poached eggs and bacon.

Nutrition: calories 270, fat 8g, fiber 2g, carbs 8g, protein 37g

SEAFOOD

23. Garlic Butter Salmon

Preparation Time: 10 minutes

Cooking Time: 15 minutes

Servings: 2

Ingredients

- 2 salmon fillets, skinless
- 1 tsp minced garlic
- 1 tbsp. chopped cilantro
- 1 tbsp. unsalted butter
- 2 tbsp. grated cheddar cheese
- Seasoning:
- ½ tsp salt
- ¼ tsp ground black pepper

Directions:

1. Turn on the oven, then set it to 350 degrees F, and let it preheat.

2. Meanwhile, taking a rimmed baking sheet, grease it with oil, place salmon fillets on it, season with salt and black pepper on both sides.

3. Stir together butter, cilantro, and cheese until combined, then coat the mixture on both sides of salmon in an even layer and bake for 15 minutes until thoroughly cooked.

4. Then Turn on the broiler and continue baking the salmon for 2 minutes until the top is golden brown.

5. Serve.

Nutrition: 128 Calories; 4.5 g Fats; 41 g Protein; 1 g Net Carb; 0 g Fiber;

24. Salmon Sheet pan

Preparation Time: 10 minutes

Cooking Time: 20 minutes

Servings: 2

Ingredients

- 2 salmon fillets
- 2 oz. cauliflower florets
- 2 oz. broccoli florets
- 1 tsp minced garlic
- 1 tbsp. chopped cilantro
- Seasoning:
- 2 tbsp. coconut oil
- 2/3 tsp salt
- ¼ tsp ground black pepper

Directions:

1. Turn on the oven, then set it to 400 degrees F, and let it preheat.

2. Place oil in a small bowl, add garlic and cilantro, stir well, and microwave for 1 minute or until the oil has melted.

3. Take a rimmed baking sheet, place cauliflower and broccoli florets in it, drizzle with 1 tbsp. of coconut oil mixture, season with 1/3 tsp salt, 1/8 tsp black pepper and bake for 10 minutes.

4. Then push the vegetables to a side, place salmon fillets in the pan, drizzle with remaining coconut oil mixture, season with remaining salt and black pepper on both sides and bake for 10 minutes until salmon is fork-tender.

5. Serve.

Nutrition: 450 Calories; 23.8 g Fats; 36.9 g Protein; 5.9 g Net Carb; 2.4 g Fiber;

25. Bacon wrapped Salmon

Preparation Time: 5 minutes

Cooking Time: 10 minutes

Servings: 2

Ingredients

- 2 salmon fillets, cut into four pieces
- 4 slices of bacon
- 2 tsp avocado oil
- 2 tbsp. mayonnaise
- Seasoning:
- ½ tsp salt
- ½ tsp ground black pepper

Directions:

1. Turn on the oven, then set it to 375 degrees F and let it preheat.
2. Meanwhile, place a skillet pan, place it over medium-high heat, add oil and let it heat.
3. Season salmon fillets with salt and black pepper, wrap each salmon fillet with a bacon slice, then

add to the pan and cook for 4 minutes, turning halfway through.

4. Then transfer skillet pan containing salmon into the oven and cook salmon for 5 minutes until thoroughly cooked.

5. Serve salmon with mayonnaise

Nutrition: 190.7 Calories; 16.5 g Fats; 10.5 g Protein; 0 g Net Carb; 0 g Fiber;

26. Stir-fry Tuna with Vegetables

Preparation Time: 5 minutes;

Cooking Time: 15 minutes

Servings: 2

Ingredients

- 4 oz. tuna, packed in water
- 2 oz. broccoli florets
- ½ of red bell pepper, cored, sliced
- ½ tsp minced garlic
- ½ tsp sesame seeds
- Seasoning:
- 1 tbsp. avocado oil
- 2/3 tsp soy sauce
- 2/3 tsp apple cider vinegar
- 3 tbsp. water

Directions:

1. Take a skillet pan, add ½ tbsp. oil and when hot, add bell pepper and cook for 3 minutes until tender-crisp.

2. Then add broccoli floret, drizzle with water and continue cooking for 3 minutes until steamed, covering the pan.

3. Uncover the pan, cook for 2 minutes until all the liquid has evaporated, and then push bell pepper to one side of the pan.

4. Add remaining oil to the other side of the pan, add tuna and cook for 3 minutes until seared on all sides.

5. Then drizzle with soy sauce and vinegar, toss all the ingredients in the pan until mixed and sprinkle with sesame seeds.

6. Serve.

Nutrition: 99.7 Calories; 5.1 g Fats; 11 g Protein; 1.6 g Net Carb; 1 g Fiber;

27. Chili-glazed Salmon

Preparation Time: 5 minutes

Cooking Time: 10 minutes

Servings: 2

Ingredients

- 2 salmon fillets
- 2 tbsp. sweet chili sauce
- 2 tsp chopped chives
- ½ tsp sesame seeds

Directions:

1. Turn on the oven, then set it to 400 degrees F and let it preheat.
2. Meanwhile, place salmon in a shallow dish, add chili sauce and chives and toss until mixed.
3. Transfer prepared salmon onto a baking sheet lined with parchment sheet, drizzle with remaining sauce and bake for 10 minutes until thoroughly cooked.
4. Garnish with sesame seeds and Serve.

Nutrition: 112.5 Calories; 5.6 g Fats; 12 g Protein; 3.4 g Net Carb; 0 g Fiber;

28. Cardamom Salmon

Preparation Time: 5 minutes

Cooking Time: 20 minutes

Servings: 2

Ingredients

- 2 salmon fillets
- ¾ tsp salt
- 2/3 tbsp. ground cardamom
- 1 tbsp. liquid stevia
- 1 ½ tbsp. avocado oil

Directions:

1. Turn on the oven, then set it to 275 degrees F and let it preheat.
2. Meanwhile, prepare the sauce and for this, place oil in a small bowl, and whisk in cardamom and stevia until combined.
3. Take a baking dish, place salmon in it, brush with prepared sauce on all sides, and let it marinate for 20 minutes at room temperature.

4. Then season salmon with salt and bake for 15 to 20 minutes until thoroughly cooked.

5. When done, flake salmon with two forks and then serve.

Nutrition: 143.3 Calories; 10.7 g Fats; 11.8 g Protein; 0 g Net Carb; 0 g Fiber;

VEGETABLES

29. Sautéed Crispy Zucchini

Preparation Time: 15 minutes

Cooking Time: 10 minutes

Servings: 4

Ingredients:

- 2 tablespoons butter
- 4 zucchini, cut into ¼-inch-thick rounds
- ½ cup freshly grated Parmesan cheese
- Freshly ground black pepper

Directions:

1. Place a large skillet over medium-high heat and melt the butter.
2. Add the zucchini and sauté until tender and lightly browned, about 5 minutes.

3. Spread the zucchini evenly in the skillet and sprinkle the Parmesan cheese over the vegetables.

4. Cook without stirring until the Parmesan cheese is melted and crispy where it touches the skillet, about 5 minutes.

5. Serve.

Nutrition: Calories: 94 Fat: 8g Protein: 4g Carbs: 1g Fiber: 0g

Net Carbs: 1g Fat 76 Protein 20 Carbs 4

30. Mushrooms with Camembert

Preparation Time: 5 minutes

Cooking Time: 15 minutes

Servings: 4

Ingredients:

- 2 tablespoons butter
- 2 teaspoons minced garlic
- 1 pound button mushrooms, halved
- 4 ounces Camembert cheese, diced
- Freshly ground black pepper

Directions:

1. Place a large skillet over medium-high heat and melt the butter.
2. Sauté the garlic until translucent, about 3 minutes.
3. Sauté the mushrooms until tender, about 10 minutes.
4. Stir in the cheese and sauté until melted, about 2 minutes.

5. Season with pepper and serve.

Nutrition: Calories: 161 Fat: 13g Protein: 9g Carbs: 4g Fiber: 1g

Net Carbs: 3g Fat 70 Protein 21 Carbs 9

31. Pesto Zucchini Noodles

Preparation Time: 15 minutes

Cooking Time: 10 minutes

Servings: 4

Ingredients:

- 4 small zucchini, ends trimmed
- ¾ cup Herb Kale Pesto (here)¼ cup grated or shredded
- Parmesan cheese

Directions:

1. Use a spiralizer or peeler to cut the zucchini into "noodles" and place them in a medium bowl.
2. Add the pesto and the Parmesan cheese and toss to coat.
3. Serve.

Nutrition: Calories: 93 Fat: 8g Protein: 4g Carbs: 2g Fiber: 0g

Net Carbs: 2g Fat 70 Protein 15 Carbs 8

32. Golden Rosti

Preparation Time: 15 minutes

Cooking Time: 15 minutes

Servings: 8

Ingredients:

- 8 bacon slices, chopped
- 1 cup shredded acorn squash
- 1 cup shredded raw celeriac
- 2 tablespoons grated or shredded Parmesan cheese
- 2 teaspoons minced garlic
- 1 teaspoon chopped fresh thyme
- Sea salt
- Freshly ground black pepper
- 2 tablespoons butter

Directions:

1. In a large skillet over medium-high heat, cook the bacon until crispy, about 5 minutes.

2. While the bacon is cooking, in a large bowl, mix together the squash, celeriac, Parmesan cheese, garlic, and thyme. Season the mixture generously with salt and pepper, and set aside.

3. Remove the cooked bacon with a slotted spoon to the rosti mixture and stir to incorporate.

4. Remove all but 2 tablespoons of bacon fat from the skillet and add the butter

5. Reduce the heat to medium-low and transfer the rosti mixture to the skillet and spread it out evenly to form a large round patty about 1 inch thick.

6. Cook until the bottom of the rosti is golden brown and crisp, about 5 minutes.

7. Flip the rosti over and cook until the other side is crispy and the middle is cooked through, about 5 minutes more.

8. Remove the skillet from the heat and cut the rosti into 8 pieces

9. Serve.

Nutrition: Calories: 171 Fat: 15g Protein: 5g Carbs: 3g Fiber: 0g

Net Carbs: 3g Fat 81 Protein 12 Carbs 7

SOUPS & STEWS

33. Cauliflower Curry Soup

Preparation Time: 15 minutes

Cooking Time: 26 minutes

Servings: 4

Ingredients:

- 2 tablespoons avocado oil
- 1 white onion, chopped
- 4 garlic cloves, chopped
- ½ Serrano pepper, seeds removed and chopped
- 1-inch ginger, chopped
- ¼ teaspoon turmeric powder
- 2 teaspoons curry powder
- ½ teaspoon black pepper
- 1 teaspoon salt
- 1 cup of water
- 1 large cauliflower, cut into florets

- 1 cup chicken broth
- 1 can unsweetened coconut milk
- Cilantro, for garnish

Directions:

1. Place a saucepan over medium heat and add oil to heat.
2. Add onions to the hot oil and sauté them for 3 minutes.
3. Add garlic, Serrano pepper, and ginger, then sauté for 2 minutes.
4. Add turmeric, curry powder, black pepper, and salt. Cook for 1 minute after a gentle stir.
5. Pour water into the pan, then add cauliflower.
6. Cover this soup with a lid and cook for 10 minutes. Stir constantly.
7. Remove the soup from the heat and allow it to cool at room temperature.
8. Transfer this soup to a blender and purée the soup until smooth.
9. Return the soup to the saucepan and add broth and coconut milk. Cook for 10 minutes more and stir frequently.

10.   Divide the soup into four bowls and sprinkle the cilantro on top for garnish before serving.

Nutrition: Calories: 342 Fat: 29.1g Total carbs: 18.3g Fiber: 5.5g Protein: 7.17g

34. Asparagus Cream Soup

Preparation Time: 15 minutes

Cooking Time: 22 minutes

Servings: 6

Ingredients:

- 4 tablespoons butter
- 1 small onion, chopped
- 6 cups low-sodium chicken broth
- Salt and black pepper, to taste
- 2 pounds (907g) asparagus, cut in half
- ½ cup sour cream

Directions:

1. Place a large pot over low heat and add butter to melt.
2. Add onion to the melted butter and sauté for 2 minutes or until soft.
3. Add chicken broth, salt, black pepper, and asparagus.

4. Bring the soup to a boil, then cover the lid and cook for 20 minutes.

5. Remove the pot from the heat and allow it to cool for 5 minutes.

6. Transfer the soup to a blender and blend until smooth.

7. Add sour cream and pulse again to mix well.

8. Serve fresh and warm.

Nutrition: Calories: 138 Fat: 10.5g Total carbs: 10.2g Fiber: 3.5g Protein: 5.9g

35. Red Gazpacho Cream Soup

Preparation Time: 15 minutes

Cooking Time: 20 minutes

Servings: 10

Ingredients:

- 1 large red bell pepper, halved
- 1 large green bell pepper, halved
- 2 tablespoons basil, freshly chopped
- 4 medium tomatoes
- 1 small red onion
- 1 large cucumber, diced
- 2 medium spring onions, diced
- 2 tablespoons apple cider vinegar
- 2 garlic cloves
- 2 tablespoons fresh lemon juice
- 1 cup extra virgin olive oil
- Salt and black pepper, to taste
- 1¼ pounds (567 g) feta cheese, shredded

Directions:

1. Preheat the oven to 400°F (205°C) and line a baking tray with parchment paper.
2. Place all the bell peppers in the baking tray and roast in the preheated oven for 20 minutes.
3. Remove the bell peppers from the oven. Allow to cool, then peel off their skin.
4. Transfer the peeled bell peppers to a blender along with basil, tomatoes, red onions, cucumber, spring onions, vinegar, garlic, lemon juice, olive oil, black pepper, and salt. Blend until the mixture smooth.
5. Add black pepper and salt to taste.
6. Garnish with feta cheese and serve warm.

Nutrition: Calories: 248 Fat: 21.6g Total carbs: 8.3g Fiber: 4.1g Protein: 9.3g

36. Beef Taco Soup

Preparation Time: 15 minutes

Cooking Time: 24 minutes

Servings: 8

Ingredients:

- 2 garlic cloves, minced
- ½ cup onions, chopped
- 1 pound (454 g) ground beef
- 1 teaspoon chili powder
- 1 tablespoon ground cumin
- 1 (8-ounce / 227-g) package cream cheese, softened
- 2 (10-ounce / 284-g) cans diced tomatoes and green chilies
- ½ cup heavy cream
- 2 teaspoons salt
- 2 (14½-ounce / 411-g) cans beef broth

Directions:

1. Take a large saucepan and place it over medium-high heat.
2. Add garlic, onions, and ground beef to the soup and sauté for 7 minutes until beef is browned.
3. Add chili powder and cumin, then cook for 2 minutes.
4. Add cream cheese and cook for 5 minutes while mashing the cream cheese into the beef with a spoon.
5. Add diced tomatoes and green chilies, heavy cream, salt and broth then cook for 10 minutes.
6. Mix gently and serve warm.

Nutrition: Calories: 205 Fat: 13.3g Total carbs: 4.4g Fiber: 0.8g Protein: 8.0g

37. Creamy Tomato Soup

Preparation Time: 15 minutes

Cooking Time: 30 minutes

Servings: 4

Ingredients:

- 2 cups of water
- 4 cups tomato juice
- 3 tomatoes, peeled, seeded and diced
- 14 leaves fresh basil
- 2 tablespoons butter
- 1 cup heavy whipping cream
- Salt and black pepper, to taste

Directions:

1. Take a suitable cooking pot and place it over medium heat.
2. Add water, tomato juice, and tomatoes, then simmer for 30 minutes.
3. Transfer the soup to a blender, then add basil leaves.

4. Press the pulse button and blend the soup until smooth.

5. Return this tomato soup to the cooking pot and place it over medium heat.

6. Add butter, heavy cream, salt, and black pepper. Cook and mix until the butter melts.

7. Serve warm and fresh.

Nutrition: Calories: 203 Fat: 17.7g Total carbs: 13.0g Fiber: 5.6g Protein: 3.7g

38. Creamy Broccoli and Leek Soup

Preparation Time: 5 minutes

Cooking Time: 25 minutes

Servings: 4

Ingredients:

- 10 oz. broccoli
- 1 leek
- 8 oz. cream cheese
- 3 oz. butter
- 3 cups water
- 1 garlic clove
- ½ cup fresh basil
- salt and pepper

Directions:

1. Rinse the leek and chop both parts finely. Slice the broccoli thinly.
2. Place the veggies in a pot and cover with water and then season them. Boil the water until the broccoli softens.

3. Add the florets and garlic, while lowering the heat.

4. Add in the cheese, butter, pepper, and basil. Blend until desired consistency: if too thick use water; if you want to make it thicker, use a little bit of heavy cream.

Nutrition: Calories: 451 kcal Fats: 37 g Protein: 10 g Carbs: 4 g

39. Chicken Soup

Preparation Time: 25 minutes

Cooking Time: 80 minutes

Servings: 4

Ingredients:

- 6 cups water
- 1 chicken
- 1 medium carrot
- 1 yellow onion
- 1 bay leaf
- 1 leek
- 2 garlic cloves
- 1 tbsp. dried thyme
- ½ cup white wine, dry (no, not for drinking)
- 1 tsp. peppercorns
- salt and pepper

Directions:

1. Peel and cut your veggies. Brown them in oil in a big pot.

2. Split your chicken in half, down on the middle. Pour water and spices in the pot. Let it simmer for one hour.

3. Take out the chicken save the meat, and toss away the bones.

4. Put the meat back in the pot, and let it simmer on medium heat for 20-25 minutes again, while seasoning to your liking.

Nutrition: Calories: 145 kcal Fats: 12 g Carbs: 1 g Protein: 8 g

40. Greek Egg and Lemon Soup with Chicken

Preparation Time: 5 minutes

Cooking Time: 30 minutes

Servings: 4

Ingredients:

- 4 cups water
- ¾ lbs. cauli
- 1 lb. boneless chicken thighs
- 1/3 lb. butter
- 4 eggs
- 1 lemon
- 2 tbsps. fresh parsley
- 1 bay leaf
- 2 chicken bouillon cubes
- salt and pepper

Directions:

1. Slice your chicken thinly and then place in a saucepan while adding cold water and the cubes

and bay leaf. Let the meat simmer for 10 minutes before removing it and the bay leaf.

2. Grate your cauli and place it in a saucepan. Add butter and boil for a few minutes.

3. Beat your eggs and lemon juice in a bowl, while seasoning it.

4. Reduce the heat a bit and add the eggs, stirring continuously. Let simmer but don't boil.

5. Return the chicken.

Nutrition: Calories: 582 kcal Carbs: 4 g Fats: 49 g Protein: 31 g

DESSERTS

41. Carrot Cake

Preparation time: 10 minutes

Cooking time: 47 minutes

Servings:6

Ingredients:

- Cooking oil spray, for greasing
- 3 eggs
- 4 ounces unsalted butter, melted
- 3 tablespoons low-carb sweetener, divided
- 2 teaspoons vanilla extract
- 2 cups grated or shredded carrots
- ⅓ cup chopped walnuts (optional)
- 1 cup almond flour
- 2 teaspoons pumpkin pie spice
- 2 teaspoons baking powder
- 1½ cups water

- 5 ounces cream cheese, room temperature

Directions:

1. Grease an 8-by-2-inch cake pan that fits in the pot with the cooking oil spray.

2. In a large bowl, use a hand mixer to beat the eggs, butter, 2 tablespoons of sweetener, and vanilla extract. Add the carrots and walnuts (if using) and stir to combine. Add the almond flour, pumpkin pie spice, and baking powder and stir until everything is combined. Pour the batter into the prepared cake pan.

3. Place the water in the pot. Place the reversible rack in the pot, making sure it is in the steam position. Place the pan on the rack. Assemble the pressure lid, making sure the pressure release valve is in the SEAL position.

4. When pressure cooking is complete, quick release the pressure by moving the pressure release valve to the VENT position. Carefully remove the lid when the unit has finished releasing pressure.

5. Carefully remove the cake from the pot. Let cool completely before frosting.

6. While the cake is cooling, place the cream cheese and remaining 1 tablespoon of sweetener in a medium bowl. Using a hand mixer, beat until the frosting is nice and fluffy. Once the cake has cooled, spread the frosting all over the top. Serve immediately or refrigerate until ready to serve.

Nutrition: Calories: 352; Total Fat: 32g; Total Carbohydrates: 8g; Fiber: 2g; Net Carbs: 6g; Protein: 8g; Erythritol Carbs: 6g Macronutrients: Fat: 82%; Protein: 9%; Carbs: 9%

42. Vanilla Custard

Preparation time: 5 minutes

Cooking time: 16 minutes

Servings: 4

Ingredients:

- 4 eggs
- ½ cup sugar substitute (like Swerve, Monk fruit sweetener, or stevia)
- 2 cups heavy (whipping) cream
- 1 teaspoon vanilla extract or 1 vanilla bean pod, split lengthwise and scraped with a knife
- Unsalted butter, room temperature, for greasing ramekins
- 1½ cups water

Directions:

1. In a large bowl, beat the eggs. Add the sweetener, heavy cream, and vanilla and whisk to combine.

2. Grease 4 ramekins with the butter. Divide the custard mixture among the ramekins.

3. Place the water in the pot. Place the reversible rack in the pot, making sure it is in the steaming position. Carefully place the ramekins on the rack. Assemble the pressure lid, making sure the pressure release valve is in the SEAL position.

4. Select PRESSURE and set to HIGH. Set time to 7 minutes. Select START/STOP to begin.

5. When pressure cooking is complete, quick release the pressure by moving the pressure release valve to the VENT position. Carefully remove the lid when the unit has finished releasing pressure.

6. Using oven mitts, carefully remove the ramekins. Let the custards cool slightly before serving, or refrigerate until ready to serve.

Nutrition: Calories: 480; Total Fat: 48g; Total Carbohydrates: 4g; Fiber: 0g; Net Carbs: 4g; Protein: 8g; Erythritol Carbs: 12g Macronutrients: Fat: 90%; Protein: 7%; Carbs: 3%

43. Vanilla Berry Meringues

Preparation Time: 15 minutes

Cooking Time: 1 hour and 45 minutes

Servings: 10

Ingredients:

- 1 teaspoon vanilla extract
- 3 tablespoons freeze-dried mixed berries, crushed
- 3 large egg whites, at room temperature
- 1/3 cup Erythritol
- 1 teaspoon lemon rind

Directions:

1. In a mixing bowl, stir the egg whites until foamy. Add in vanilla extract, lemon rind, and Erythritol; continue to mix, using an electric mixer until stiff and glossy.

2. Add the crushed berries and mix again until well combined. Use two teaspoons to spoon the meringue onto parchment-lined cookie sheets.

3. Bake at 220 degrees F for about 1 hour 45 minutes.

Nutrition: 51 Calories 0g Fat 4g Carbs 12g Protein 0.1g Fiber

44. Hazelnut Cake Squares

Preparation Time: 10 minutes

Cooking Time: 25 minutes

Servings: 8

Ingredients:

- 2 cups almond meal
- 3 eggs
- 1 teaspoon almond extract
- 3/4 cup heavy cream
- A pinch of sea salt
- 1/2 cup coconut oil
- 1/2 cup hazelnuts, chopped
- 3/4 teaspoon baking powder
- 1 cup Erythritol
- 1/2 teaspoon ground cinnamon
- 1/4 teaspoon ground cardamom

Directions:

1. Set the oven to 365°F. Coat the bottom of your baking pan using parchment paper.

2. Thoroughly combine the almond meal, baking powder, Erythritol, cinnamon, cardamom, and salt.

3. After that, stir in the coconut oil, eggs, almond extract, and heavy cream; whisk until everything is well incorporated.

4. Stir in the chopped hazelnuts. Scrape the batter into the baking pan.

5. Bake in the oven for at least 25 minutes.

Nutrition: 241 Calories 23.6g Fat 3.7g Carbs 5.2g Protein 1g Fiber

45. Espresso Pudding Shots

Preparation Time: 10 minutes + chilling time

Cooking Time: 0 minutes

Servings: 6

Ingredients:

- 2 teaspoons butter, softened
- A pinch of grated nutmeg
- 1 teaspoon pure vanilla extract
- 4 ounces coconut oil
- 3 tablespoons powdered Erythritol
- 4 ounces coconut milk creamer
- 1 teaspoon espresso powder

Directions:

1. Melt the butter and coconut oil in a double boiler over medium-low heat.
2. Add in the remaining ingredients and stir to combine.
3. Pour into silicone molds.

Nutrition: 218 Calories 24.7g Fat 1.1g Carbs 0.4g Protein 0.7g Fiber

46. Cinnamon Raspberry Smoothie

Preparation Time: 11 minutes

Cooking Time: 0 minutes

Servings: 1

Ingredients:

- 1 cup of unsweetened almond milk
- 1/2 cup of frozen raspberries
- 1 cup of spinach or kale
- 1 tbsp. of almond butter
- 1/8 tsp of cinnamon, or more to taste

Directions:

1. Place all the ingredients into the blender and blend until pureed.
2. Enjoy as breakfast or snacks.

Nutrition: 286 calories 21g fat 19g carbohydrates 10g protein

47. Bulletproof Coffee

Preparation Time: 5 minutes

Cooking Time: 0 minutes

Servings: 1

Ingredients:

- 2 tbsp. MCT oil powder
- 2 tbsp. Ghee/butter
- 1.5 cup Hot coffee

Directions:

1. Empty the hot coffee into your blender.
2. Pour in the powder and butter. Blend until frothy.
3. Enjoy in a large mug.

Nutrition: Protein Count: 1 gram Total Fat Content: 51 grams Net Carbohydrates: 0 grams Calorie Count: 463

48. Peanut Butter Caramel Milkshake

Preparation Time: 5 minutes

Cooking Time: 0 minutes

Servings: 1

Ingredients:

- 2 tbsp. Natural peanut butter
- 1 tbsp. MCT Oil
- .25 tsp. Xanthan gum
- 1 cup Coconut milk
- 7 Ice cubes
- 2 tbsp. Sugar-free salted caramel syrup

Directions:

1. Combine each of the components in a blender.
2. Mix thoroughly and serve in a chilled mug.

Nutrition: Protein Count: 8 grams Total Fat Content: 35 grams Net Carbohydrates: 5 grams Calorie Count: 365

49. Chocolate Shakes

Preparation Time: 10 minutes

Cooking Time: 0 minutes

Servings: 2

Ingredients:

- 4 oz. Coconut milk
- .75 cup Heavy whipping cream
- 1 tbsp. Swerve natural sweetener
- .25 tsp. Vanilla extract
- 2 tbsp. Unsweetened cocoa powder

Directions:

1. Empty the cream into a cold metal bowl. Use your hand mixer and chilled beaters to form stiff peaks.
2. Slowly add the milk into the cream. Add in the rest of the fixings.
3. Stir well and pour into two frosty glasses. Chill in the freezer one hour before serving. Stir several times.

Nutrition: Protein Count: 4 grams Total Fat Content: 47 grams Net Carbohydrates: 7 grams Calorie Count: 210

50. Strawberry Almond Smoothie

Preparation Time: 10 minutes

Cooking Time: 0 minutes

Servings: 2

Ingredients:

- .25 cup Frozen unsweetened strawberries
- 2 tbsp. Whey vanilla isolate powder
- .5 cup Heavy cream
- 16 oz. Unsweetened almond milk
- Stevia (as desired)

Directions:

1. Toss or pour each of the fixings into a blender.
2. Puree until smooth.
3. Pour a small amount of water to thin the smoothie as needed.

Nutrition: Protein Count: 15 grams Total Fat Content: 25 grams Net Carbohydrates: 7 grams Calorie Count: 34